618.9    Bryant, Jennifer.
BRY
         Sharon Oehler,
           pediatrician.

                         33197000039193

$15.95

| DATE | | | |
|------|------|------|------|
| 11-22 | | | |
| 1-17 | | | |
| 2-9 | | | |
| | | | |
| | | | |
| | | DISCARDED | |
| | | | |
| | | | |
| | | | |
| | | | |
| | | | |
| | | | |

BAKER & TAYLOR BOOKS

# Sharon Oehler:
## Pediatrician

Published by
Twenty-First Century Books
38 South Market Street
Frederick, Maryland 21701

Text Copyright © 1991
Jennifer Bryant

Photographs Copyright © 1991
Pamela Brown

Printed in the United States of America

10 9 8 7 6 5 4 3 2 1

Cover and book design by Terri Martin

*Dedicated to all of the working moms
who helped with this project*

Library of Congress Cataloging in Publication Data

Bryant, Jennifer
Sharon Oehler: Pediatrician

Summary: Portrays the everyday life of a hard-working pediatrician who is
also a busy mother raising a family.
1. Oehler, Sharon—Juvenile literature. 2. Pediatricians—United States—
Biography—Juvenile literature. 3. Working mothers—United States—Juvenile
literature.
[1. Oehler, Sharon. 2. Physicians. 3. Working mothers.]
I. Brown, Pamela 1950- ill. II. Title. III. Series: Working Moms.
RJ43.O34B79   1991   618.92'00092—dc20 [92]   90-24370 CIP  AC
ISBN 0-941477-53-3

# Sharon Oehler: Pediatrician

Jennifer Bryant
Photographs by Pamela Brown
Photographic Consultant: Bill Adkins

TWENTY-FIRST CENTURY BOOKS
FREDERICK, MARYLAND

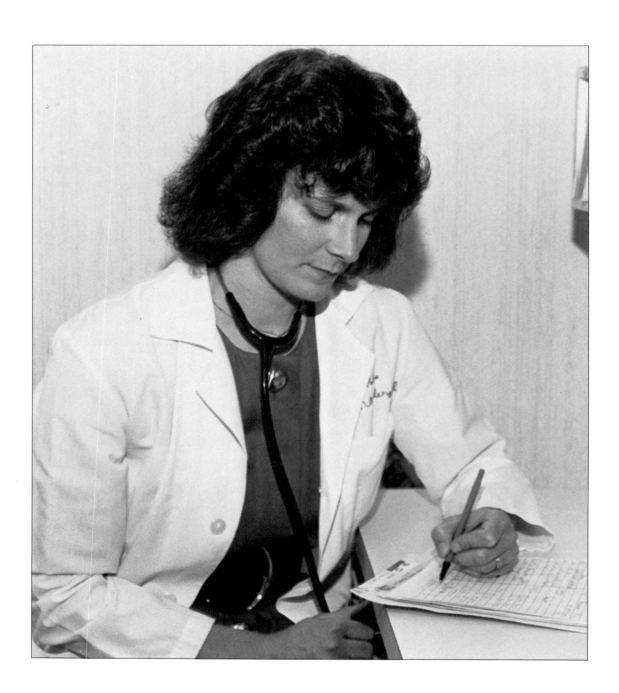

"Chester County Hospital Staff Only!" reads the sign at the entrance to the parking lot. Sharon Oehler quickly finds a parking space close to the hospital. "Now why can't I ever find a spot like this during the day?" she wonders.

It's 2 o'clock in the morning. Only minutes ago, Sharon had been at home, fast asleep. Suddenly, she was awakened by the ringing of the phone. "Please come right away," the nurse on duty at the hospital requested. "Mrs. Grimes' baby is ready to be delivered."

Sharon was awake at once. After all, this was not the first time she had been called to work in the middle of the night. Dr. Sharon Oehler is a pediatrician, a doctor who takes care of children. And, as Sharon knows, children don't always wait for the morning to need a doctor.

It didn't take long for Sharon to get dressed (even in the dark) and say a silent good-bye to her sleeping family—to her husband Dan and three daughters, Amanda, Breanna, and Abbie. "It's hard to leave my family like this," Sharon thinks, "but now Mrs. Grimes is starting a family of her own—and I need to be there."

"It's just part of the job," Sharon reminds herself. "It's part of being a working mom."

A pediatrician is the kind of doctor you probably go to when you get sick. Sometimes, a pediatrician has to be present when a newborn baby is delivered. Mrs. Grimes' baby is going to be born through a special operation called a Cesarean section (or "C" section, for short). And it's Sharon's job to make sure that the newborn baby is healthy.

"Off to a good start"—that's what Sharon says she wants for each of her newborn patients.

At the hospital, Sharon hurriedly climbs the stairs to the second floor, where the maternity ward is located. This is the area where pregnant women deliver their babies. Before she can help with Mrs. Grimes' delivery, however, Sharon has to "scrub up," or wash her arms and hands. She wants to be sure that she doesn't carry any germs into the delivery room that could infect Mrs. Grimes or the newborn baby.

Sharon puts on her "scrubs," the long, green pants and shirt that doctors and nurses wear. And she slips on a new pair of clean, plastic gloves. Now Sharon takes a deep breath and enters the delivery room. Mrs. Grimes has been prepared for surgery, and Mr. Grimes—dressed in scrubs, too—is close by her side.

It's 2:20 A.M.

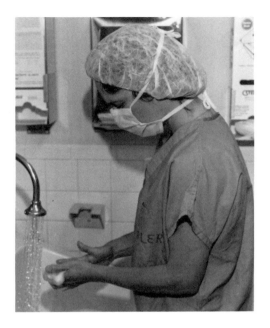

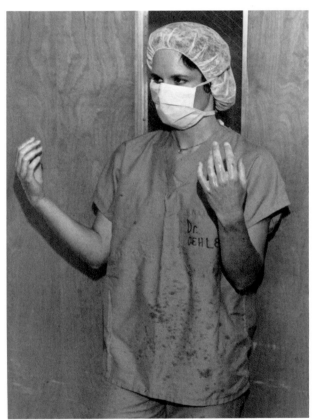

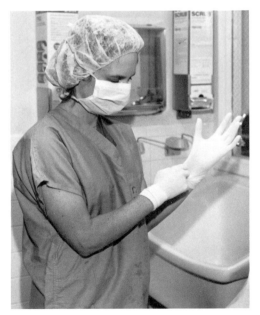

At 3:13 A.M., Mrs. Grimes' baby, a girl, is born. Sharon uses a suction hose to clear out the baby's mouth, throat, and breathing passages. The hose removes any mucus—a thick, sticky fluid—that might make it hard for the baby to breathe. When Sharon removes the hose from the baby's mouth, Mrs. Grimes' little girl lets out a big cry.

Now Sharon and the nurses give the baby a quick check-up to make sure that she's off to that "good start." "She looks good," one of the nurses says to Sharon, who checks the baby's heart and lungs. Sharon agrees: "She looks fine, Mrs. and Mr. Grimes." Sharon hands the baby to one of the nurses. Her work tonight is finished. Another baby is off to a good start.

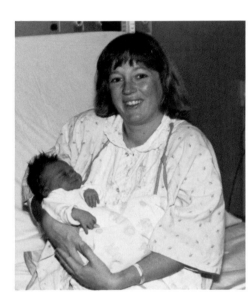

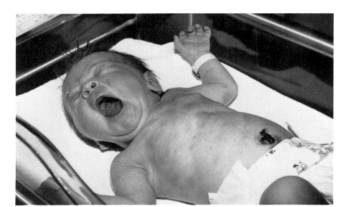

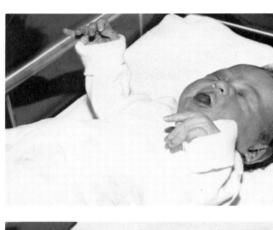

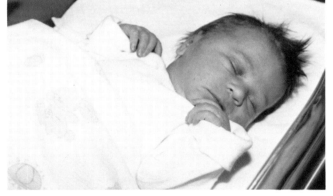

As the Grimes meet their new daughter, Sharon removes her scrubs and washes up. "I never get tired of watching babies come into the world," Sharon thinks. "It's truly a miracle. Each time I see a healthy newborn, I realize how lucky I am to have such a rewarding job."

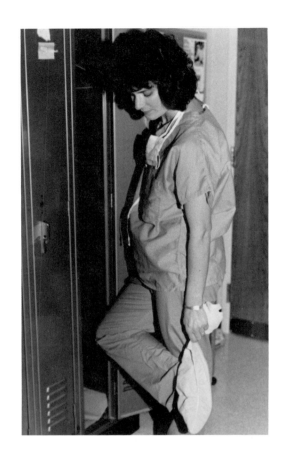

For a moment, Sharon turns her thoughts to the Grimes. She knows that having a baby changes so many things. Sharon remembers when her first baby, Amanda, was born. At that time, Sharon was studying and training to be a doctor, working more than 100 hours a week and sometimes staying at the hospital around the clock. "The decision to start a family was not an easy one," Sharon recalls. "I wasn't sure that Dan and I could handle all of the responsibility."

Sharon knows that being a working mom is not easy. At times, it seems that being a doctor, a wife, and the mother of three children is too much for one person to do. At times, it seems that it's too much for one person to be.

"But whenever I feel overwhelmed," Sharon says, "I remember my grandmother. She raised a family while working as a full-time teacher. And she did it in the days when there were no microwave ovens, disposable diapers, dishwashers, or washing machines. It must have been tough, but she managed to do everything without complaining."

Sharon's grandmother set a good model for her daughter and her daughter's daughter. "It was from my grandmother," Sharon says, "that my mother learned this attitude. I guess that's where I get it from, too. My brother and sisters are all hard workers. It's just the way we were raised. It's a good way, I think."

It's 4:00 A.M.: Sharon has to be back at the hospital in just a few hours. She could sleep on one of the cots set aside for doctors, but Sharon decides to go home. Even if it means getting a little less sleep, she wants to see her family when they wake up in the morning.

"Still, I hate giving up this parking space," she laughs.

It's quiet as Sharon slides back under the warm covers. She takes a quick look at the clock. The glowing face of the clock reads 4:30 A.M.

"Mom, Mom! It's time to get up," seven-year-old Breanna shouts as she pushes open the door to her parents' room. The clock says 6:30 A.M., and the two hours of sleep feel more like two minutes. "May I wear shorts today?" asks Breanna. "Is it going to be hot or cold?"

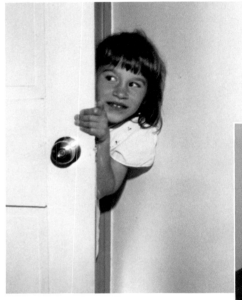

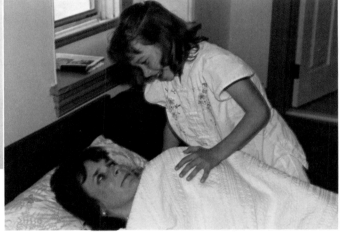

"Thanks for the wake-up call, Breanna," Sharon replies. She rubs her sleepy eyes. "Yes, you may wear shorts today," she tells Breanna. "But not your new ones. Save them for our big trip." Next week, the family's going on a vacation to Yellowstone National Park.

Sharon shakes her head as she watches her middle daughter disappear down the hallway. "I've only been awake for 30 seconds, and I'm already a working mom," she thinks, throwing off the covers. She starts to get dressed for the second time this day.

"What's that wonderful smell coming from the kitchen?" Sharon asks herself. But she already knows the answer. "I'd recognize the smell of Dan's famous pancakes anywhere!" Dan is a project director for an engineering company. Like Sharon, he chose a profession that requires a lot of time and energy.

Before leaving the bedroom, Sharon opens the windows to let in the fresh air of this new day. The first two windows open easily, but the third one is stuck. Sharon pushes against the window frame with all of her might, but it doesn't budge an inch. "Darn!" she complains. "There's another project to add to our 'fix-it' list. Sometimes I think that list will never stop growing!"

"Our friends thought Dan and I were crazy to buy this big, old house," Sharon remembers. "They didn't think we'd find the time to fix up this place. It did need a lot of work. But we did a little painting, a little wallpapering, a little refinishing each weekend. And slowly, very slowly, it's become our home. We're still working on it. And the girls help, too. It's one of our favorite family activities."

In the kitchen, the three girls are busy helping their father make breakfast. Amanda, who's ten, sets the table while Breanna gets out the orange juice and maple syrup. Dan hands four-year-old Abbie a stack of pancakes on a serving plate. "Be careful with these, Abbie," Dan cautions. "They're still hot."

Her sisters watch eagerly as Abbie brings the pile of steaming pancakes to the table. Amanda and Breanna both reach for the one on top. Their father has made it in the shape of a mouse!

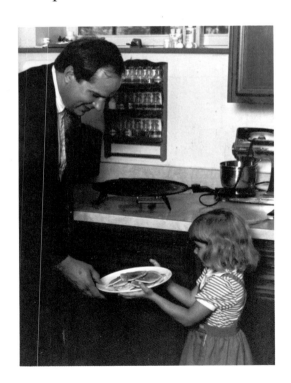

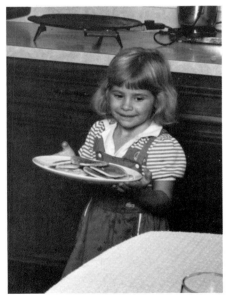

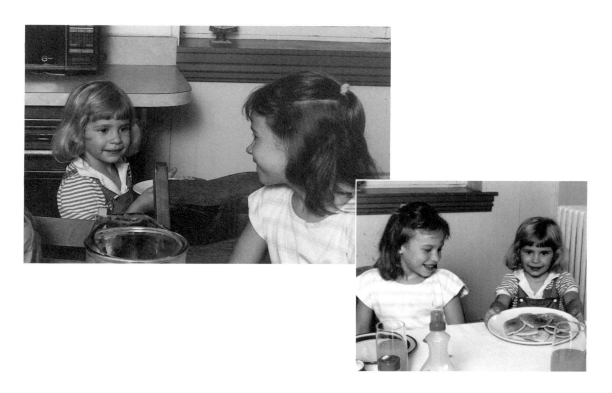

"Hey, this one's mine," declares Amanda. "I asked Dad to make it for me!"

"But I had my fork in it first!" replies Breanna.

"All right, girls, there's certainly enough for everyone," Sharon says as she enters the room. "You two can split that one and take one more each to start."

"I get the ears," Amanda insists.

"Well, I want the tail," says Breanna. "It tickles when you eat it."

Today, as on most school days, the children help clean up after breakfast. Sharon packs lunches while Dan helps Abbie get ready for the day ahead. The two older girls go to school on the bus, and Dan takes Abbie to nursery school on his way to work.

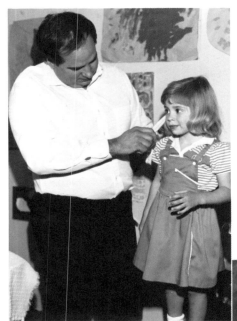
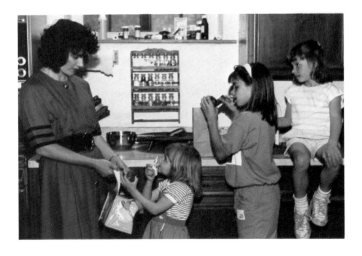
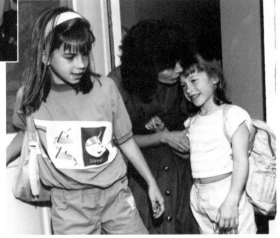

It's 7:15 A.M.: everyone is out the door. Sharon returns to the hospital for her morning "rounds," a series of daily visits to check on her patients. She checks on her newest patients first. "Good morning," she says to the nurse on duty at the nursery, the part of the hospital for newborn babies. "What have we got today?"

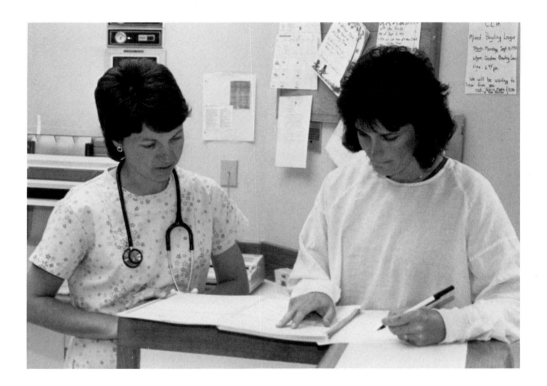

"Seven new little people," the nurse answers.

"That's not too bad," Sharon replies. She can remember mornings when there were 30 newborns or more.

Sharon's first patient today is a seven-pound boy. He was born two days ago. Wearing a white hospital gown, Sharon examines the baby carefully. He doesn't seem too happy about it.

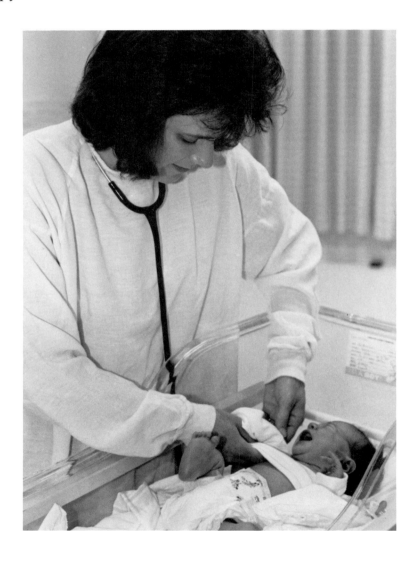

She measures the baby's weight and length.

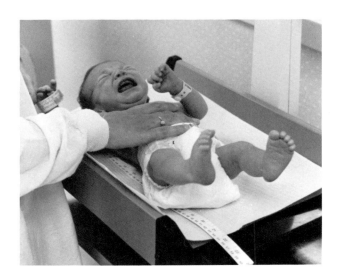

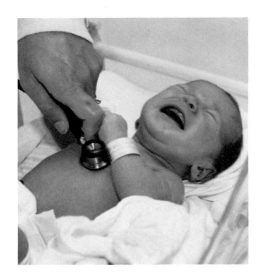

She uses a stethoscope to listen to his heart rate and breathing. She checks to see that his pulse is strong and that his lungs are clear of mucus.

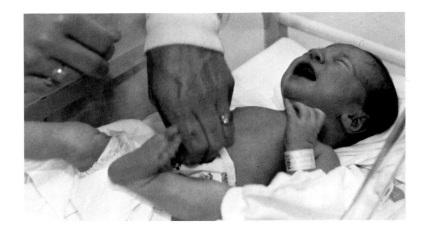

She unfastens his diaper and looks at the umbilical cord. (This is the cord that connected the baby to his mother during pregnancy.) Sharon wants to make sure that the cord is healing normally.

She checks the baby's hips by moving his knees apart and back together. Sharon sees that the baby's hips are not out of joint.

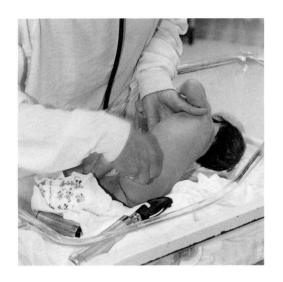

She uses an otoscope to look into the baby's throat and ears.

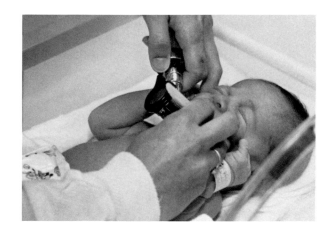

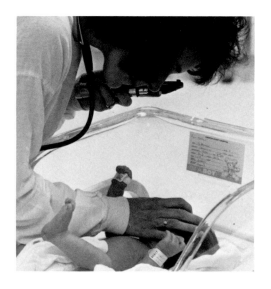

She studies the baby's eyes with an ophthalmoscope, an instrument that tests his response to light.

"This baby looks fine," Sharon reports to the head nurse when the newborn check-up is over. "He can go home today."

The second baby that Sharon examines today seems to have a faint, yellowish look. "It's probably a slight case of jaundice," Sharon notes. Jaundice is a condition of the blood system that causes the skin and body fluids to look yellow. Sharon explains: "It's a fairly common problem and usually not serious. We put these babies under a special light, and in just a day or two, the skin color is fine and they can go home."

Next, Sharon's rounds take her to a premature infant. Sometimes called a "preemie," a premature baby is one that's born sooner than expected. "Some of these babies need extra care," Sharon says, "because their bodies are not quite ready to work on their own. If they are too weak to suck, they may need to be fed from a tube that sends food directly into the bloodstream. Or if they have trouble breathing on their own, they may receive oxygen from a machine called a ventilator."

The premature baby girl that Sharon sees today was born four weeks ago. (She was born about eight weeks before the mother's "due date," the date when the mother was expected to deliver her baby.) Sharon listens to the baby's lungs and is pleased to hear her strong and regular breathing. "She's almost ready to be taken off the ventilator," Sharon says to the head nurse. Then she whispers to her little patient, "Just a few more days and you'll be on your own."

After the babies are examined, it's time to see the mothers. Sharon tries to answer all of their questions about baby care. And they do have lots of questions, especially the new mothers! How often should the baby be fed? How do I know when the baby is hungry? ("They'll let you know," Sharon tells the worried mothers.) What do I do if the baby gets diaper rash? Is it okay to use a pacifier? Is my baby's head shaped funny?

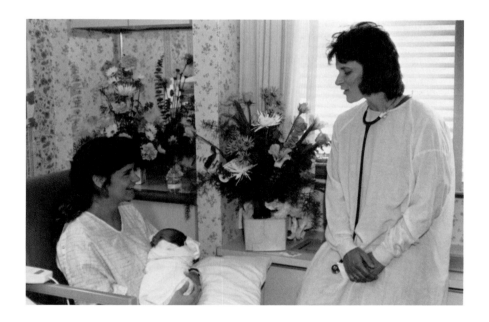

Sharon gives each new mother a quick lesson in baby care. "Just as important," she explains, "I try to reassure these new mothers that they are going to do just fine. Right now, they have the new-mother jitters. I can remember how that felt."

When the morning rounds are over, Sharon goes to her office for the day's appointments. Her office is just across the street, and Sharon makes a quick stop on her way to get a cup of tea at the hospital cafeteria. Enjoying a brief break from the day's hectic pace, Sharon thinks back to a time when she doubted that she'd ever "make it" as a doctor.

To become a pediatrician, Sharon took many college science courses, including biology, chemistry, and anatomy. After college, she was accepted to medical school. That meant four more tough years of school ahead. The first two years were spent mostly in laboratories and classrooms, learning more about science and medicine. The last two years were "rotations"—going to different hospitals and learning about the many different kinds of medicine, called specialties, that doctors practice.

This was a very important time for Sharon and the other students in her class. It was their opportunity to decide what kind of doctor they would become. Those who wanted to specialize in treating children would become pediatricians.

For Sharon, the choice was easy. "I first thought about becoming a children's doctor when I was in elementary school. I grew up with some children who had serious health problems. I remember thinking, 'Somebody should be able to help these kids.' Much later, in medical school, after getting some real experience with sick children, I knew I wanted to become a pediatrician."

Sharon was one of only 30 women in a medical school class of 250 students. But she never let that discourage her. "My parents had brought me up to do my best, and I was confident that my best would be good enough," she says.

But it wasn't easy. And it didn't get any easier when, in the last year of medical school, Sharon had her first baby girl.

"There were days when I was so tired I could hardly stand up," Sharon recalls. "The other students were tired, too, but they didn't have a baby to take care of when they got home. But that was a choice I made, and now I'm glad I did. I think having a family helped me take a more balanced approach to my work. Medical school and training were important then, but they weren't the only things that mattered. That's an attitude I still have today."

After medical school, Sharon completed a three-year pediatric "residency." During this time, she worked under the direct supervision of several pediatricians. The women pediatricians were especially good role models for Sharon. In addition to their demanding jobs, many of them had families to take care of, too. Their example helped give Sharon the confidence she needed to become a good doctor. "I figured if they could do it, so could I!" Sharon says.

And she did. Now Sharon practices medicine with four other doctors at West Chester Pediatrics. The sign on the front of her office shows the result of years of hard work: "Sharon Oehler, M.D.": Sharon Oehler, Medical Doctor.

Over the years, West Chester Pediatrics became well known in the community. As the medical practice grew, Sharon's family was growing, too. Sharon and Dan had two more children and continued to balance (they call it "juggling") the demands of work and family.

In the course of all these changes, they tried different types of child care. Doctors have unpredictable schedules—medical emergencies can happen anytime, day or night. But most of the day-care centers and baby sitters had regular "9 to 5" hours. "If I had an emergency at the hospital and Dan was needed at his office, I'd be in a real panic trying to find someone to take care of the children," Sharon says.

Sharon and Dan decided to hire a nanny to live with them and take care of the children. That type of in-home child care worked well when their daughters were very young. Now, however, all three of the girls are in school at least part of the day. When classes are over, they attend after-school programs nearby. This gives them a chance to start their homework and visit with their friends.

Does Sharon worry about not being a "stay-at-home" mother? "No, I really don't," she says. "I've always worked outside the home, and the girls accept that. For them, it's normal to have me go to the office every day." She adds with a smile: "The other day one of Amanda's classmates said to her, 'I went to see your mom for a check-up today.' Amanda told me she's proud that I'm a doctor."

It's 10:15 A.M., and Sharon picks up the appointment schedule from her desk. It's going to be another busy day—as usual.

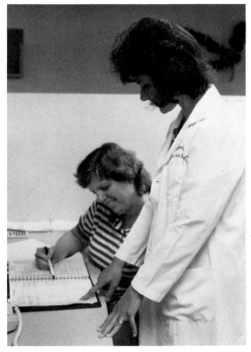

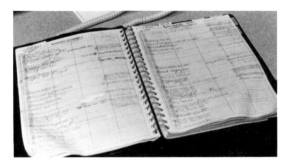

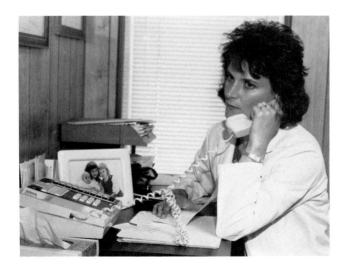

Sharon takes the time to return phone calls from worried parents. She listens carefully to their concerns. If a condition sounds serious, Sharon will ask them to bring their child to the office.

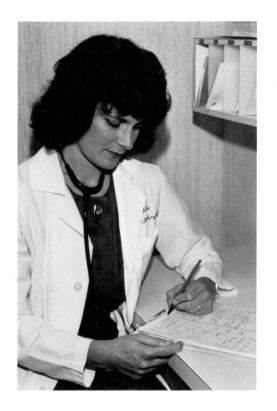

Her first appointment is with three-year-old Melissa Tate. First, Sharon carefully reads the medical chart that the nurse has prepared. The chart notes that Melissa has been complaining about a sore throat for the last several days.

"Good afternoon," Sharon says as she enters the room where Melissa and her mother are waiting. Sharon asks Melissa's mother when the soreness was first noticed, whether Melissa has been running a fever, and whether there are any other symptoms to report. A symptom is a warning sign that some part of your body is not working in a healthy or normal way. It may be a fever or an upset stomach. It may be pain, redness, or swelling. Doctors must pay close attention to a patient's symptoms. They are the clues that help a doctor find out what is wrong.

"How are you feeling today?" Sharon asks Melissa.

"My throat hurts," Melissa complains.

Sharon examines Melissa's throat and ears. She is looking for any signs of infection. An infection is a disease that is caused by germs that have invaded the body. Sharon is looking for any signs of strep throat, an infectious disease caused by germs called bacteria. It's the kind of disease you can "catch" from someone else. If Melissa has strep throat, she'll need a medicine called an antibiotic to help her body fight the germs that are making her sick. But Sharon doesn't see the redness and swelling that come with strep throat.

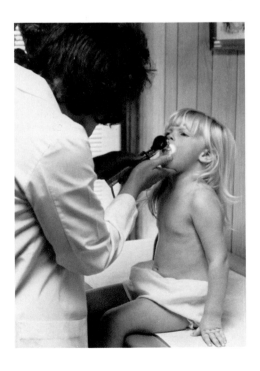
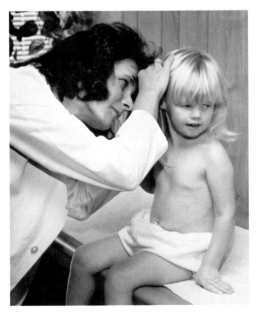

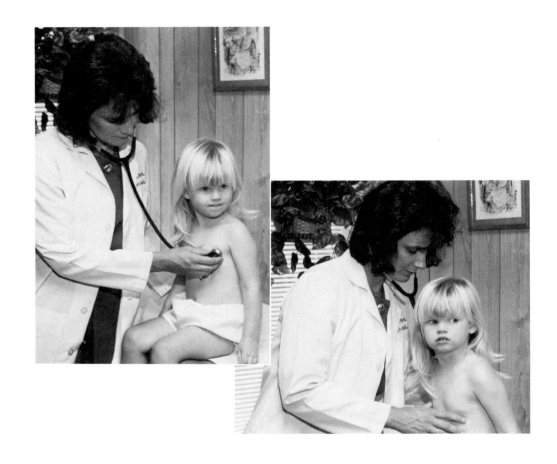

   Next, Sharon gives Melissa a general check-up. "It doesn't look serious," Sharon reports to Mrs. Tate. "It's probably just a cold." A cold is an infectious disease, too, but it is caused by germs called viruses. The best way to get over a cold is to get plenty of rest and drink lots of fluids. "But if Melissa isn't better by the end of the week," Sharon continues, "please call. We may have to take another look."

Mrs. Tate thanks Sharon, and Melissa waves good-bye as she leaves the examining room. Sharon switches on the mini tape recorder that she carries in her pocket. Speaking slowly and clearly, she records important information about Melissa's office visit.

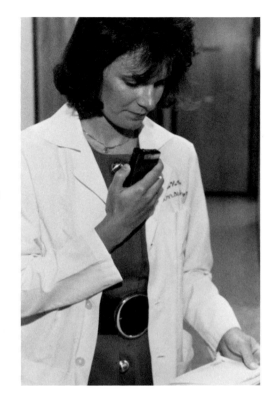

"It's very important for a doctor to keep clear and accurate records for each patient and each appointment," Sharon observes. "I used to write this information on the patient's chart after each appointment. But it took too much time. So now I use the tape recorder. Then, at the end of each day, the secretary listens to my recording, types out the information on the patient's record, and places the written record in the patient's folder. This way, I stay on schedule with my appointments."

Staying on schedule is not as easy as it sounds. Sharon's afternoon is filled with a variety of patients and problems.

Ryan Cobb is here for his regular six-month check-up. Mrs. Cobb says, "He's growing up so quickly." And Sharon smiles because she knows that feeling so well.

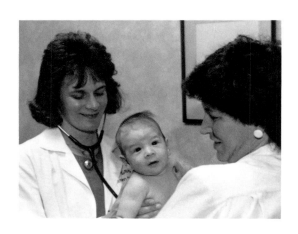

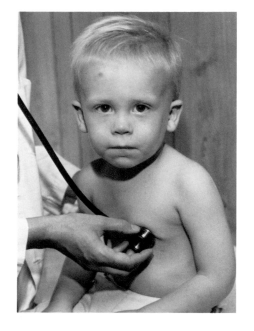

Three-year-old Mark Corey has a cough and a tight feeling in his chest. "Well, let's just check this out," Sharon says to Mark, who doesn't seem to be too happy about his visit to the doctor.

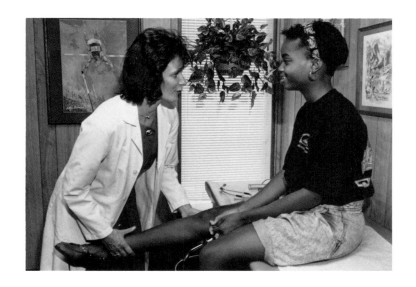

Thirteen-year-old Tamara Smith is here for a physical, a general examination of her health, so that she can play soccer for her middle-school team. "You're in great shape," Sharon announces. "Good luck with the team!"

Steven Maitlin is six years old and has just started swimming lessons. "He's been having earaches," his mother explains. "Should I keep him out of the water?"

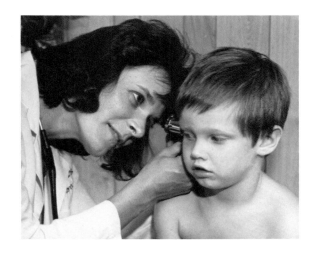

Sharon sees patients until 5 o'clock. It's a long and tiring day, but the day isn't over yet. Now it's time for Sharon to pick up her youngest daughter from school. Abbie is busy playing at the nursery school as Sharon drives up. "Mommy, today we had a picnic in the park," Abbie exclaims. "It was really fun."

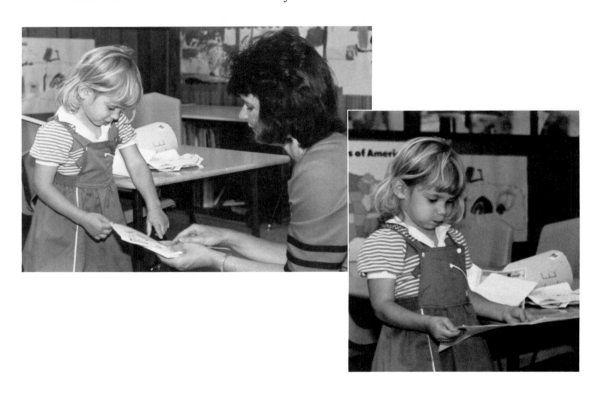

As Sharon pulls out of the school's driveway into the heavy, rush-hour traffic, Abbie gives her mother a lengthy and breathless account of everything that happened to her at school today.

Sharon likes to listen to Abbie's adventures. But she's also thinking about the things that have to be done tonight—working on the house, helping the girls with their homework, giving Abbie a bath. There's laundry to do and bills to pay. "Thank goodness Dan is cooking dinner tonight!" she thinks.

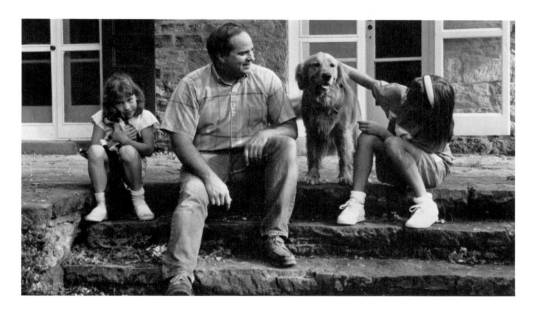

Dan, Amanda, and Breanna are sitting on the front steps when Sharon and Abbie arrive at the house. "Hey, Mom, you'll never guess what we saw on the bus ride home today," Amanda says. Sharon smiles a tired smile and gives her husband a tired hug.

"Why don't you tell her about it at the dinner table?" Dan wisely suggests.

"Okay," Amanda replies, leading her two sisters inside to the kitchen.

"How was your day?" Sharon asks her husband.

"It was fine," Dan says. "But I found out that we've got another project to do on the west coast. I'll have to fly out there for a week."

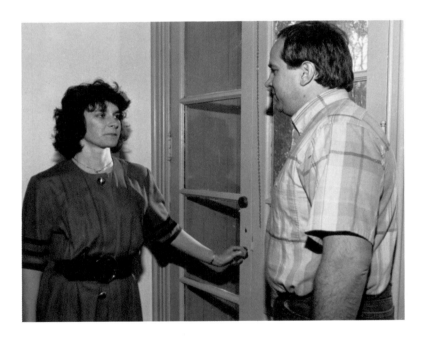

Already, Sharon begins thinking about the child-care arrangements she'll have to make while Dan is gone. But that has to wait. Right now, there's meat loaf to be eaten and children's stories to be heard. Around the dinner table everyone joins hands to give thanks for their health and their family.

As Sharon uncovers the meat loaf, the girls begin to giggle. Dan has made it in the shape of a bear!

"We knew you'd be tired tonight," Dan says cheerfully, "so the girls and I wanted to remind you that vacation's not far away!"

"I get the arms," Amanda shouts.

"Can I have the nose?" asks Breanna.

Sharon laughs and asks for a big piece. "You know," she says, "I think I'm going to enjoy seeing bears instead of babies for a while."

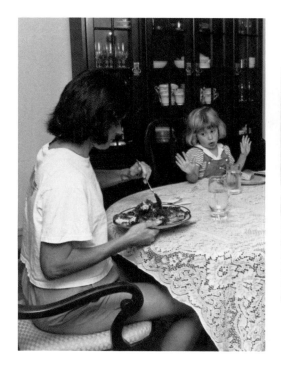
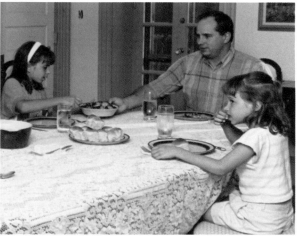

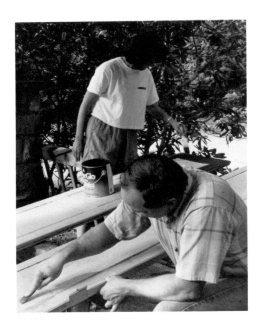

After dinner, Sharon and Dan often work on one of the projects on their ever-growing fix-it list. In the last light of the evening, they repair the house's old shutters. If the girls get their homework finished in time, they'll get to put on the final coat of paint.

"Working on this old house is a family hobby," Sharon says. This spring, Dan and Sharon made a new swing for the back porch. "Now when a long day is over, we can sit back for a few minutes and enjoy a quiet moment together. It's a good way to end the day."

But tomorrow is certain to be another busy day, so it's time to put work away and get the girls in bed. Then it's time to clean the kitchen and do the laundry. And Sharon wants to finish sewing a doll blanket for Abbie's birthday.

"Put work away?" Sharon asks herself. "Not much chance of that. Whether I'm at the office, at the hospital, or at home, I'm always a working mom."

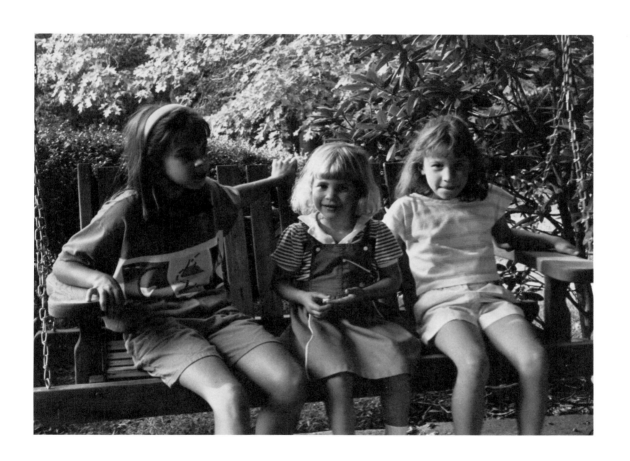

# Glossary

| | |
|---|---|
| **antibiotic** | a medicine used to stop the growth of harmful germs |
| **Cesarean ("C") section** | a special operation sometimes needed to deliver a baby |
| **check-up** | a routine medical examination |
| **due date** | the date a pregnant woman is expected to have her baby |
| **germs** | tiny living things that cause infectious diseases |
| **infection** | when the body is invaded by disease-causing germs |
| **infectious disease** | a sickness that can spread from one person to another |
| **maternity ward** | the part of the hospital where pregnant women deliver their babies |
| **nursery** | the part of the hospital where newborn babies are kept |
| **ophthalmoscope** | an instrument used to check the eyes |
| **otoscope** | an instrument used to check the throat and ears |
| **pediatrician** | a doctor who takes care of children |
| **pediatrics** | the kind of medicine that deals with children |
| **physical** | a general medical examination |
| **premature baby** | a baby who is born much sooner than expected |
| **symptom** | a warning that the body is not working in a healthy way |
| **stethoscope** | an instrument used to listen to sounds within the body |
| **ventilator** | a machine that helps premature infants to breathe |